EXERCISE HACKS

Table of Contents

INTRODUCTION

It's the beginning of the year, which means new goals and resolutions, fresh minds but some glitches.

What is this glitch I speak of here? You may wonder

I'm speaking of your body. The man's tit is excessively grown and saggy, the woman's waist is becoming significantly large and floppy, and the beer belly is looking like a bag of pruno.

The arms? Oh no!

It's quite similar to a shoestring. Not only that, some tend to have a large stomach with upper back fat or body fat in the lower body, the lower legs; whichever one you have, don't get me wrong, I'm not body shaming anyone. We all look unique with our different body sizes and all, no doubt about that, but you know you would look better if there were no excesses in your arm, stomach, and other areas, all of which can make you look unfit. You can bet that a fit but a sexy body, irrespective of your size, is an eye-catcher, and we all want to have that kinda body.

Have you got these excesses? If yes! Amazing. So that you know, you are not alone.

I've always had the same fat-ass problem until I learned the hacks outlined in this book. So, don't stop reading yet.

These hacks are effective, and they helped me keep fit. If it did me, so it would you.
These hacks would make you have a SWOL body, looking fit at just five minutes for the first day and one minute more every workout day after that!
Since I've got your attention now, let me briefly introduce who I am before moving into the book proper.

The name is Big Rome; you see the Big in the title, that's to tell you I was quite famous for my body size. Anyways, I was born and raised in the late 80s in Salinas, California, a tough little town with a high murder rate. I was a good kid, and I was also sociable and ended up being a class clown, but I also got into a fair share of trouble, which of course, eventually got me behind walls.

Through all that Hogwash, I learned some of the best exercises that require no weight lifting, and I can bet you're going to love it.
Writing to you now, after about an hour of engaging in these hacks, I am sweat dripping, breathing hard, slight sore in my Legs, core, chest, arms, shoulders, and all that.

For starters, it might hurt a little more, and it's quite understandable but do note that apart from the sores, you'd be burning some calories all in five minutes on the first day.

You don't believe me yet? Follow me, guys. I'm about to change your life and build your body structure into getting capabilities substantially!
As a bonus, you might even learn how to conduct yourself like a real g along the way!

Winks

Now here is the problem with most of us.
We all want to lose some pounds, get in shape before the year runs out, or preferably we want to become sexier so we can show off some abs and muscle to family and friends during Thanksgiving or to our crushes during a date.

Whichever reason you have, losing weight is a great and exciting thing. However, the problem begins not with the wishes and goals but with having to "do," i.e., giving up a few minutes each day and putting in the efforts to achieve that fitness goal we have set up for the year.

Do you know why this is a problem?
 It's because WE'RE LAZY

Don't roll your eyes! That's the blunt truth.

We all are. No more, no less.
Like if there were some awards for being lazy, we'd still send in someone to collect such recognition while we remain in pajamas at home.

From one excuse to the other, we end up providing reasons and excuses that suit all seasons, all the time.

I can't jog because it's cold outside.
It's too hot to run now; I might get sunburns.
I don't have gym wear.
Blah, Blah, Blah

I wasn't the type who gave excuses or who wanted to lift the remote control up and down ten times, wipes off beads of sweat just like Catriona Harvey Jenner once quoted in her blog.
Nah, I wasn't.

I've had my first share of exercises early in life. As stated earlier, I was growing up being chubby and not in the best shape, and as such, at the age of 14, I couldn't even do one push-up. I hated being fat so much that I had to sign up for an exercise routine, gave it all I got until there's nothing left, but it's better not to take more than 15 minutes because I often hated doing long, boring exercises.

So just like me, these long exercises bore me out, but this book, having the hacks, is like a silver lining that will show you ways to reduce your body excesses within a little minute more than five.
Just like the famous saying, it's the minor changes you adopt and maintain (the five or more minutes of engaging in these hacks) that generally add up to a meaningful long-term difference.

Enjoy the book but put in the effort!

CHAPTER ONE: CAN'T I JUST DO NOTHING?

I don't feel like exercising today. Can't I do nothing?

Do nothing to burn calories? Nada!

It isn't the first time you're saying this; it was the same yesterday, the day before, and a few weeks ago, and it most likely won't be the last, but you should know it's in your best interest that you engage in exercises. I know your head's not in the game because you are an award-winning Lazy person, but being lazy doesn't mean you should do nothing. If you want to improve your physical self, then chances are you're frequently exercising; five minutes for the first day and more minutes for every other day.

The truth about being Lazy is that you are not always going to feel like training all week, all the time; however, you need to be a grown-up about these things and do the stuff you don't feel like doing. No doubt you don't like doing anything, but you might need to make yourself do it anyway.

You know exercise is good for you, the health benefits of regular exercise are too hard to ignore. Maybe you are lazy because you do not see how good exercises are in your life in general.

Let's have a little glimpse into some of the benefits of exercises that can lead to a happier, healthier you.

- **Weight Control**

Engaging in exercises, no matter how little, has a way of increasing your metabolic rate, which will burn calories and prevent you from getting excess weight gain while you also maintain a loss. The more intense the activity, the more calories you burn, and if you can't find a large chunk of time to exercise every day, don't worry; any amount of activity is better than none at all.

- **Health Risks Reduction**

Irrespective of your current weight, engaging in exercises tends to keep your blood flowing smoothly. When your blood flows smoothly to every organ in your body, there's a tiny chance of experiencing heart disease, stroke, diabetes, or high blood pressure. However, if you're already suffering from these health problems, regular exercises help you manage them from escalating.

As blood flows smoothly to every part of your body, it delivers oxygen and other nutrients to make your system, energizing it, so it works more. With increased energy, you'll have more strength to take on more chores or tasks.

- **Mood Booster**

Need an emotional lift from depression, stress, and anxiety?
Then there you have it. Regular exercises stimulate the release of happy hormones, which produces positive feelings and improves your mood, leaving you feeling more comfortable, more relaxed, and less anxious. Irrespective of the intensity of the workout, your mental state benefits from exercises
As you begin these hacks consistently, you'd also end up feeling better about your appearance; this gives a boost to your confidence as well as your self-esteem.

- **Better Sleep**

Regular exercises not only enable you to fall asleep faster, but it also deepens your sleep and makes you get better sleep.

- **Spark in the Bedroom**

Everyone loves sex, but it's not something anyone will look forward to if it's boring. If you are out of shape or too tired, you'd not enjoy intimacy to its fullest, which can be frustrating for both genders.

However, when you engage in exercises, it releases several hormones, which causes arousal in women and reduces erectile dysfunction in men.

- **Morale Booster**

Often workout sessions help to boost your morale and make you a little stronger. Once you are into a minute of your workout routine, you'll find the inner strength to keep doing it. Regardless of age, sex, or physical abilities, you'd find yourself having the drive to keep burning calories.

These are just a few out of the numerous benefits of engaging in exercises. Once you begin these hacks and become consistent with them, you'd improve your life.

Consistency is key! Follow the options in this book because they are significant steps to burn those calories without visiting the gym.
So, get your lazy fat ass off the couch and workout today!

CHAPTER TWO: HACK I (STRETCHES)

Now you've perfectly understood the dangers of not exercising at all: from heart disease, stroke, diabetes, to boring sex life. That's the more reason why you should workout, no matter how little.

You can do these hacks in whatever way; they can also be incorporated effectively into your daily lives so quickly and at your convenience. You do not need a whole room to yourself for this; just a corner is okay.

You should note that if you engage in these workout hacks for up to 10 minutes per day, that equals 60 hours of exercise per year, excluding other physical activities you have to do, like doing the chores, climbing the stair, etc. If you can move these hacks from ten minutes per day to twenty, i.e., after the five minutes on the first day, then you'd be moving your body and making it more robust and better for 120 hours a year.

Isn't that easy and amazing?

The primary thing is starting. Start small and feel good; it will be beneficial not just in your health but also in other vital areas of your life. So, oh ye couch potatoes, and let's begin.

Easy Stretches For "Laziest"

We'd begin with stretches. No doubt, this is not one of the most exciting parts of working out, but stretches will help you improve flexibility, reduce any form of stiffness or tightness, and eventually, make your workouts enjoyable, more efficient, and safer; without injury or pain. Whatever we'd be doing will help maintain and improve the length of our muscles from every undue strain. Now let's get started and warm up with stretches.

Stretch One

Stand straight with your legs side by side, then you clasped your hands together at the center of your chest, with your palm laid on each other. Then stretch slowly up and down for a couple of seconds. With each stretch, you'd be warming up your arms, shoulders, and chest.

Stretch Two

Stand straight but with your fingers interlaced at your back and pull your body downwards with your neck bent down towards the back. It will enlarge your respiratory passageways, arms, and shoulders.

Stretch Three

Stand straight with a clasped hand lifted high above your head. Then you stretch upwards, and you can also extend a little to the back.

Stretch Four

Lay your right knee flat on the floor, on your exercise mat, or any soft objects while the left knee should be lunged forward in front of you (90 degrees). It would help if you still bent the right leg underneath you. With hands-on your waist, slightly push hips forward with your hands and stretch. It would be best if you did it for each knee.

You could also place both hands on top of your right knee and press your back hip forward, leaning into the stretch, but keep your torso upright. Hold for 30 seconds; release. Do three reps; switch legs and repeat.

Stretch Five

Lay on your mat with one leg raised. Now use an item of lengthy clothing, e.g., a towel, to hold your feet up in the air and stretch. It would help if you did it for both legs.

Stretch Six

Bend your right elbow to the back so your right hand can touch the top middle of your back. Stretch out your left-hand overhead to grasp just below your right elbow. Then you gently pull your right elbow down and toward your head after a few seconds. Switch arms and repeat. You can do this while kneeling, standing, or sitting.

Notes

You may or may not do all these stretches, but you shouldn't stop at just one. As you engage in these stretches, you should inhale and breathe out as you stretch your arms, waist, and upper body in whatever direction.

After warming up for a couple of minutes, it's time to increase our heart rate and burn off a few calories. You could either skip or jog in a place at your pace. When doing each of these activities, keep it easy; you're neither in a competition or are you to be chase down by a cop. Do either of them for some minutes and stop when you can tell your heart rate has increased.

CHAPTER THREE: EXERCISE HACK II

Though we struggle to make time for engaging in exercises, these hacks will help keep the body fit rather than just lying on the bed and doing nothing. Though it feels good to sit in front of the television and eat a pack full of Ores, you'd be doing your body a lot better by doing these easy workouts.

Now let's move to the second segment of the hacks. After the stretches, which are quite good for the hip, arms, thighs, and back, we'll engage in much more strenuous activity, so you can burn more calories and preferably get some abs. Do not fret! They are relatively easy, and I'd advise you to stick to one routine for a couple of seconds, sweat out, and begin the following exercise.

Remember, if today is your first, you'd be doing this for five minutes alone but some minutes more for subsequent days, and believe me, you might end up doing much more than you imagine. That's the beauty of exercises.

These hacks would work majorly on your arms, legs, abdomens, back muscles, abs, and for the women, butt, and legs.

Now let's go!

Modified Push Ups and Planks

Not able to do the complete pushups? Here are modified easy ways to do it and get the same results.

Routine One

Stand with your feet jointly, then lay on your mat with your palms flattened on the floor to lift your weight. Now push yourself off the floor to a considerable height, then stand up and bend your knees before going back to the floor. I understand perfectly if this is too hard to do, but if you can do this twice or thrice on the first day, then you'd do more as the week rolls by. Don't go hard on yourself.

Routine Two

I'll call this the Superman Plank because it is how he flies, but we are not doing the whole of it because we've got no superpowers. Here we go:

Now assume a plank position on your mat but make sure your body is straight and supported by your toes and forearms. After you've taken this position, then you gradually lift your left arm and your right leg, then you hold for at least three seconds (for starters). It would help if you did this movement for the right arm and the left leg.

After doing twice of this in a set (i.e., the left arm and right leg), I'd suggest you go for a squat before resuming for the next batch (i.e., the right arm and left leg). The squat will enable you to catch your breathe in-between this routine.

Routine Three

Bend to the floor and stay in that high plank position, but rather than raising yourself entirely, you'd break the routine at your knees.
That is, you'd bend your elbows to lower your upper body toward the ground to do a complete push-up, but you'd drop to your knees and walk your hands together so that your thumbs and forefingers form a triangle. Then you'd stand back up to be sure you're stepping on one leg at a time, so it's easy on the back. Do this five or ten times, then do ten to fifteen squares immediately after for one set.

Routine Four

This routine is similar to the pattern we just finished. The only difference is that you'd do two full push-ups before squatting five or ten times. That is, for one set, ten or twenty push-ups would be followed by ten to twenty squats immediately after. Make sure you use a chair or couch as a low point to step at when squatting; you can sit properly and stand back up but be sure you keep your legs, knees, and back straight and pretend there's a bar glued to your knees so they don't wobble left to right.

Routine Five

This routine includes five push-ups; then, you'd get up
and do five squats for one set. Each workout's goal is ten
sets but don't overwhelm yourself if you can only do one
or two sets. Just do it every day, and eventually, you
won't get tired after that first or second set; you're likely
going to do more! Being consistent will ignite a fire in
your heart, and you'll know you are on your way to being
the epitome of health!

Benefits

The above workout routines are quite beneficial for your
flappy arms that wave back. Am I quite sure your arms are
presently burning? That's progress. Now stay with me;
these routines are all designed to help with your posture
and body strength while aiding stability. Let's move onto
the next.

Forearms and Back Routines

Routine One

Following a routine is quite similar to squatting, but this is a lot easier. Get a chair without an arm or a couch seat, a keg, whatever about your knee height; stand with your feet hip-width apart in front of the chair. Now keep your arms by your side and gradually lower yourself into the chair with your hands clasped. Your back should be straight as you lower your thighs into the chair. Do this repeatedly for a couple of more seconds as this routine helps you work on your core and lower body.

If sitting on a chair isn't okay for you, then you can sit against the wall too! All you have to do is lean against a wall and then slide down until the legs form a 900 angle. Now, try to hold this position for a couple of seconds before getting up and repeating it.

OR

You stand in front of the chair or whatever you are using, then place your hands on the top with your fingers pointing forward. Keep your back straight and bend past the seat towards the floor while walking your legs out in front of you until you're in a somewhat sitting position. As you lean towards the floor, your elbows should directly be behind your body but should straighten out as you lift your body to your previous stand position. Do this for a couple of minutes.

Routine Two

Quite similar to the superman plank routine explained above. Remember, we've got no superpowers, so you'd only lie down on your mat! It isn't the time to catch a breath or fall asleep.

***You should catch your breaths in between exercises.

After lying with your face down on the mat, you'd hold out your arms to your sides at shoulder-height. While doing this, then you simultaneously lift your chest, arms, and legs off the ground while giving yourself two thumbs up with your fingers. Now hold your lifted self and feel the burn before lowering your back to the mat. Repeat this as long as you can.

Routine Three

In this routine, you'd need a piece of household equipment. Maybe a can of veggies, a water bottle but preferably a dumbbell, if you have one. Whichever you have should be placed vertically on your mat.
Now you'd begin in a high plank (i.e., push up position) with both of your hands holding onto the dumbbell resting on the floor. Then you'd pull your right elbow back slowly while lifting the dumbbell toward the chest but keeping the elbow close to the torso. Do this on each side repeatedly.

OR

If you have a friend that wants to work out with you, you both can get in a push-up position facing head to head around two feet apart; then you do a push-up, giving each other a high five with the opposite hand. Do these ten times, or you make it fun by doing it until someone quits. After this, you then hit ten squats or repeat the push-up exercise or a rematch.

Routine Four

This one can be called "navy seals." Now, do a push-up, quickly bring your left knee to your chest, and then do the same for your right knee. Now that counts as one; do these five to ten times, then get up and do some squats.

Routine Five (Optional)

These are called "jlos," but they feel good for the hamstrings. To do this, you'd put your hands to the floor with your knees bent and closed together so they can go through the arms without hitting them. After that, start moving your butt up and getting very low to the ground. I bet you can't do thirty if you're an urban beast.

Benefits

Now, these outlined routines are a great way to work on your legs, back, and arms. They help burn calories, improves body core strength and abdominal tone muscles.

Legs Routine

Routine One (Donkey Kicks)

It is one great exercise to help you lose fat fast.
Go down on all fours and make sure your hands are
placed beneath the shoulders with your palms on the
floor and knees below your hips. Now kick back with one
of your legs upwards while the other knee is bent. Do this
repeatedly on one leg before switching such movement
to the other leg.

You can also do mountain climbers such that you'd be in a
push-up position, then start with a left knee to the chest,
then right. Do as much as you can; try twenty or thirty for
one set. It can be a good exercise if you don't feel like
doing push-ups or squats but want to do something.

Routine Two (Mostly for women)

This one can be duck walks. Put your hands on your head,
and with your back straight, squat close to the ground and
stay there. Now walk in that squat position and make sure
you have room; even though you might not walk that far,
do this as many times as you can set wise. It is another
good one if you don't want to do push-ups or squats.

Routine Three

Stand with your feet wide apart, then hinge forward into
a squat. Make sure your knees are bent until your thighs

are parallel to the ground. Now leap into the air as high as you can go while straightening out your legs.

You should also swing your arms down to your sides and keep your back straight and chest lifted. Hit the floor softly with your knee bent as you go directly into another squat.

Routine Four (Lunges)

I know you might be quite aware of this cause it's one of the most popular practical exercises that can help you lose some fat. You begin with standing tall with your feet wide apart, then you place your hands on your hips and step forward with one leg (your right leg) while keeping your spine tall. Then you lower your body until the left, and your right legs assume a 90-degree position. Then you hold for three seconds before doing the same movement for the other leg.

You could also stand tall with your feet apart, then you step your left leg slantways behind your right leg and bend your knees to lower into a lunge. You then push through your left heel to stand and bring your left leg back to start. Repeat on the other side.

Routine Five

Here, do a push-up and get up as many times as possible, preferably up to ten. If you get this far, you're a beast. Now start at ten and go back to one.

Benefits

These routines target the legs, core, and chest and help you build many lean muscles. You can as well get strong legs and tight thighs by sitting! Yeah, you heard me right. Sit on a chair comfortably and do a leg raise for a couple of seconds, then do the same for the other leg or try raising your knees.

Abs Routine

Routine One

Before we start, you should know that this routine might hurt a little bit, but it's worth it, so keep going. We'd start with you, sitting on the floor with your knees bent but your feet lifted and hands behind your head. Gently lean back while keeping your chest up and back straight; now, then hold your abs tight before twisting to bring your right elbow to your left knee. Repeat this on the opposite side as well for a couple of seconds.

Routine Two

Lay on the mat in a plank position with your elbows stacked underneath your shoulders. Now, stretch your entire body forward, so your shoulders go past your elbows toward your hands, then take it back to the starting position. Look at the floor while you and continue for a few more seconds.

Routine Three

Be in that same plank position but with your hand on the floor rather than your elbow. Now draw your left knee to your right elbow while keeping your toes off the ground before returning your left foot to the starting position. Switch legs and do the same thing. Continue repeatedly for a couple of seconds.

Routine Four

Lie flat on your back with your knees bent and your hands facing downwards; then lift your hips before lowering them back to the ground. Repeat this for some seconds.

Benefits

Burn off excess fat, strengthens muscles that run along the sides of the torso, rib, and hip. The above abs hack highly effective and, if done consistently over time, will yield the tremendous results needed.

***

No doubt, your body hurt like hell!
No cause for alarm. To ease the sore and cool off, you can engage in a few simple stretches, and I can bet, but you'd feel good again.

CHAPTER FOUR: TIPS FOR KEEPING UP DAILY

It's not going to be easy working out at home and at your own time, especially when the couch is around the corner and your favorite show is never-ending, but here are a few tips on how to stay motivated.

Arrange a spot in your living room or kitchen beforehand so you won't feel lazy when you feel like working out. Get your mat ready and a bottle of water at the spot the night before if you would work out the next day. Set out your clothes the night before, so working out will be more convenient, giving you fewer excuses for why you don't have the time.

Fix a time and show up at the spot. The time should be at your convenience, and you should dress the part, i.e., you should show up in gym clothes, not in pajamas. I'm not saying you should spend a fortune getting a gym outfit, any workout outfit will do, and it is vital because you are more likely to do it if you dress the part.

Start. Just start. No matter how small, it could be two minutes or even less. Start by trying to complete at least half of five minutes.

Since you'd be starting these routines after months, if not years, of lazing around, you should not go hard on yourself, else you might find it hard getting back to these routines the next time. You don't have to be all-perfect or do the whole thing; you should do something, try it the first few seconds, take a break and continue.

Make a habit out of it; else, it won't happen. Set aside a specific time and do something, not exercise. After a few weeks, you would use your body to do something at that time, and then you can start these hacks.

Go on walks in the evening or during long phone conversations. Long walks are a great way of getting an hour of exercise during a time that you'd be doing nothing anyway.

Try to eat a snack that's high in simple carbs before you exercise because simple carbs have proven to provide your body with energy.

Track your progress by keeping a workout calendar and tick up all the days you successfully do these routines. It will motivate you to keep doing it, and in fact, it will boost your confidence as you watch the progress you're making.

Music does magic. Take time to create a few playlists filled with inspiring workout songs to prevent fatigue. You can as well follow people that will inspire you to get active on social media.

Remember not to do the stated routines at once; we're not after that. However, doing nothing is worse, and do not force yourself to do what you hate.

Finally, while you're engaged in these routines, you need also to watch your eating habits because they go hand-in-hand.